LETTERS

ON

DIPHTHERIA,

BY

J. H. PULTE, M. D.

AND

EGBERT GUERNSEY, M. D.

SAINT LOUIS, MO.:

Published by R. & H. LUYTIES,

No. 51 NORTH FIFTH STREET, BET. OLIVE & LOCUST,

(LUYTIES' HOMŒOPATHIC PHARMACY.)

Fr. Kluender, Printer,
Corner Third and Chesnut Streets,
St. Louis, Mo.

PREFACE.

For sometime past, but especially in the last twelve months, a very serious disease has prevailed with more or less fatality in the western country. This disease is called DIPHTHERIA. In consequence of its rapid and fatal termination in many cases, much anxiety is felt and expressed by the people as to the most speedy and reliable measures to be employed by them in time of necessity and danger. In order to meet this inquiry and demand for the purpose of promptly combatting this formidable disease, request was made of several physicians of much experience in this particular, to give the symptoms and treatment of this affection for public use. Dr. Pulte of Cincinnati, and Dr. Guernsey of New York, have kindly responded to the request, furnishing short treatises upon the subject which are subjoined. While our obligations are hereby acknowledged to the gentlemen named for their services in this behalf, we hope and believe the treatment recommended by them will be of incalculable value to every family and the means of saving many lives.

Respectfully,

R. & H. LUYTIES,

Proprietors Homoeopathic Pharmacy.

St. Louis, December, 1860.

DIPHTHERIA.

(AS TREATED BY DR. J. H. PULTE.)

This disease is comparatively a new one, with whose nature and character we have had heretofore but little acquaintance. It now has appeared amongst us in an epidemic form, and we have had abundant opportunities to study its character and treatment. Though dangerous, if not recognised and treated in the beginning, it admits of very successful treatment, if carefully watched and immediately met by the proper remedies. In this respect it resembles the Asiatic Cholera which also proved terrible only when neglected in the beginning or not at all recognized as such.

Diphtheria attacks all ages, but principally the Young and among these the full, fleshy children. Adults are scarcely taken with it, except by real infection from others and in such cases the results are more severe. The disease has an infectious character, but only by immediate transmission of portions of saliva or membranous shreds of the patient into the mouth, nose, eyes or wound of another; mere exhalation seems not to propagate the disease, though even in very severe cases, where the exhalations become very fetid, this may also be the case. Whether the disease attacks the same person more than once during life or the same season, is not known as yet.

Like other epidemics, which favor particular organs as places of development, it increases the frequency and danger of those diseases peculiar to those organs and impresses upon them more or less of its own character. If during Cholera times diarrhœas were very frequent and obstinate, though they were strictly speaking not real Cholera attacks, so we have now sore throats in abundance and find them more obstinate than heretofore.

DIAGNOSIS. It is already generally known that this disease principally affects the throat and many have been induced to believe that it is nothing more than a malignant form of ulceration of the throat, similar to that which accompanies the scarlet fever or appears in its stead. Others believe it to be a new species of Croup with greater extent and fatality. But those opinions are not correct. There are similarities between these diseases, because the locality of their appearance is the same; yet their differences are so great, that we must not consider them to be of the same family.

Diphtheria is a disease, the germ of which enters the system in the form of a miasm, like that of cholera or any other miasmatic disease and then in the course of its development propagates its own germ on the locality, peculiar to itself and that is the throat.

In this respect we can consider it indeed a disease of the blood, which is penetrated by its poison through and through, if by non-interference we permit it to do so; if we can check the progress of this poison or neutralize its very existence, then have we indeed cured the patient, not sooner.

The first symptom almost in every case is a subdued hoarseness, a slight huskiness in voice and apparent weakness of utterance. As this is frequently not observed, the disease progresses without any thing being done to stop its progress. In more acute cases this slight hoarseness may be quickly followed by high fever and more severe symptoms of the throat, which then invite immediate attention to the sufferer. In other cases the disease proceeds without any or much fever, so that the state of the patient is not revealed except by observing closely the changes on the tonsils and palate. There will then be seen a whitish exudation, of various size and shape, from a pin's head to a five cent piece, not like matter or pus, loose and easily to be detached, but tough, like wash-leather of a dirty white colour. In the progress of the disease, if not checked, this spot enlarges in extent and thickness, until it reaches like a white bridge from tonsil to tonsil, descending into the pharyngeal cavity, where its observation is lost to the eye. In its further progress the same exudation invades the larynx, trachea and even entering the bronchial tubes, if life has not terminated sooner by laryngeal spasms.

The most distinguishing features of the disease aside from the throat symptoms, are: Muscular weakness, showing itself mostly in a listless, lazy apathy, yet not averse to complacently noticing or even playing; paralytic appearances, such as difficult swallowing of liquids, more than solids;—difficult, rather uncertain articulation;—hollow, snoring respiration; coughing after or during an attempt to drink; loss of appetite for almost any thing to eat or drink (this is one of the most unfavorable symptoms.)

In some cases the glands of the neck and throat become involved, swell up to a fearful extent as in malignant scarlet fever and show all the symptoms of a critical suppuration; yet when the glandular abcess is opened, the condition of the vascular walls is found broken down and fatal arterial hemorrhage ensues. In other cases the disease invades the nasal fossae and a fetid mucus runs from the nostrils, corroding and obstructing the nose, similar to some cases of malignant scarlet fever. In these cases a comatose state soon supervenes and life ends under paralysis of the brain, as in the other cases, described above it ended in paralysis of the lungs.

Another fatal issue of the disease can be by a metastasis or translation to the stomach and its environs;—in such cases the throat symptoms may disappear and in their stead black vomiting ensues which soon terminates life.

We have also witnessed in two cases the following train of symptoms:

In the first case the diphtheritic characteristics disappeared in a few days; the child returned to school, but in two days thereafter complained of headache, lost sight, hearing, speech, could not smell, taste nor swallow—had great difficulty in raising the accumulated phlegm from throat or lungs, which almost terminated its life. Yet it recovered from this fearful paralytic state, but lost all the hair on its head. Its recovery was as perfect as it is usually after severe typhus fever, if no severe lesions have taken place. The other case was similar to this one, but the child being considerably younger and of feebler constitution, it died in one of those efforts to overcome the accumulation of phlegm by a sudden attack of paralysis of the brain.

These facts as to the occasional termination of the disease prove its real toxical character, similar to the most virulent of the typhus species, if induced by poisonous malaria or contagion.

This view is strengthened by issues bearing still a closer resemblance to the typhoid forms, such as petechiae and livid spots, like bruises (purpura hemorrhagica) with the attending low type of fever.

We could still produce more evidence of the essential nature of this disease as expressed above, if in a popular article of this kind, it was considered necessary. Enough is stated to convince the reader of the fearfulness of the disease and the necessity to combat it in the onset and if possible to prevent its progress; we have more power to prevent it, than to cure it.

TREATMENT.

As this treatise is intended for popular use only, we adapt its injunctions to that purpose. Professional men must follow their own experience, or if they will profit by ours, we hope they will find them well founded. We want four remedies in the possession of the reader: ACONITE, BELLADONNA, KALI CHLORICUM and BINIODIDE OF MERCURY.*

Besides these internal remedies, we recommend as a gargle a solution of salt and water, and around the throat a bandage dipped in a similar solution. If the disease commences with FEVER, give first ACONITE and BELLADONNA (five drops of each in two tumblers, half full of water) every hour a teaspoonful, until the fever subsides.

In some cases the fever subsides under this treatment in 8 or 10 hours, yet on examination of the throat, it will be found that the diphtheritic white spots have not disappeared or even diminished; in such cases as well as in those, where the fever still continues after the exhibition of ACONITE and BELLADONNA, we must hasten to exhibit the following remedies in their order and continue their exhibition, until all the throat symptoms with the fever have disappeared; this may sometimes last two or three days.

These remedies are: BELLADONNA, KALI CHLORICUM and BINIODIDE OF MERCURY; the two first in solution, five drops of BELLADONNA and twenty drops of KALI CHLORICUM, each in a separate tumbler half full of water; of the third remedy, which is in powder form, the dose for children of four years and over is so much as will lay on a three cent piece, for children under four years it is half that quantity; of the two first in liquid the dose is a teaspoonful, and half a teaspoonful respectively as to the age of the patient. The time of exhibition varies from one, two to three hours; in the beginning every hour a dose, i. e. the first hour BELLADONNA, next hour KALI CHLORICUM and the third hour the powder of BINIODIDE OF MERCURY dry on the tongue; the fourth hour BELLADONNA again and so on. If the patient is better or at least not worse next day, the time of exhibition may be lengthened to two hours and afterwards to three hours. When all the throat symptoms have disappeared, but fever is yet present more or less, the last remedy may be

* The strength or degree of these medicines is as follows: *Aconite*, first decimal in tincture; *Belladonna*, same as *Aconite*; *Kali chloricum*, in a saturated solution (1 part to 16 parts of distilled water;) *Biniodide of Mercury*, first decimal in powder.

entirely omitted and the two first may be still given until every vestige of the disease has left.

During all this time the external application of the saltwater-bandage (covered with flannel) must not be omitted for an instance; if dry it must be removed; the children, if old enough, to know how, must be directed to gargle frequently with luke-warm salt water. This latter means we also recommend as the best preventive EXTERNALLY to those exposed to the infectious influence of this disease; as INTERNAL preventive we recommend the use of a small quantity of the Biniodide of Mercury or still better of Iodide water alone every day once.

DIET. During the disease the strength of the patient should be kept up by all means possible; for this purpose we recommend broths of meat, claret-wine, wine-whey, &c.; if patients desire oysters and ice-cream, especially during convalescence it may be given to them. If possible keep them in bed in a moderately warm and even temperature. Change the linens frequently and air the rooms as often as convenient.

DIPHTHERIA.

(AS TREATED BY DR. E. GUERNSEY.)

Diphtheria, from the Greek word *διψτερα*, the prepared skin of an animal, is by no means a new disease. It prevailed as an epidemic in France more than forty years since and was admirably described by several English Authors nearly a century ago. I have met with cases in my own practice as early as 1846.

It is called diphtheria, from the tendency to the formation of a false skin or membrane in the throat. The disease I think is most decidedly a blood disease, developing itself in the throat and rapidly prostrating the vital forces. It cannot therefore be treated merely as a local trouble, but while prompt measures should be taken to arrest its ravages in the throat, the treatment must also be general. There are two kinds of DIPHTHERIA, the MILD and the SEVERE or MALIGNANT.

The disease usually sets in with vomiting of a thin fluid, oftentimes followed by purging of the same character. This is followed by prostration and a kind of stupor. In the mild form there is no fever, and these symptoms are slight, but in the more malignant cases the symptoms are not only severe and the prostration great, but the skin becomes hot, the mouth dry and feverish, and the desire for water constant, which however is thrown up almost as soon as taken. The patient does not yet complain of sore-throat, but on looking the throat presents a bright red appearence. In a short time the bright red parts begin to be covered by a whitish substance looking not like an ordinary ulcer, but like a membranous deposit thrown upon the surface. This deposit increases until it seems to fill the whole mouth and nostrils. The smell, if the disease assumes an ulcerative character, as it frequently does, is generally offensive, and sometimes blood bursts from the nostrils, or is thrown up from the ulcerated surface. The powers of life fail rapidly. The patient gasps for breath as in croup, and tears at the throat for that relief, which often alas only comes with death. In the mild cases, as I have said before, all the symptoms are slight. There is little or no fever, but the attack is almost always preceded by vomiting, and in a short time there is found in the throat on the tonsils, the membranous deposit.

A good nourishing diet and a few doses of the Bi-Chrom-Potash given every three hours, and a gargle of alum water, or Chlorate of Soda will usually suffice to effect a cure in these mild attacks.

In some cases the disease runs its course rapidly not unfrequently terminating in death in forty-eight hours. In these cases the false membrane rapidly forms, and the patient as in croup, dies from suffocation. In other cases the disease is more slow in its progress and several days may elapse before the change for convalescence or death takes place.

Treatment.—Diphtheria, although presenting many of the symptoms of Scarlatina, must not be confounded with that disease, or mistaken for the ordinary forms of ulcerated sore throat. It is not merely a local disease, although its worst and most fatal symptoms are developed in the throat. It is a disease of the blood, poisoning the entire system and rapidly prostrating the vital forces. The throat is the index, showing the march of the disease. The treatment then should be both general and local; general, to support the system, to enrich the blood and increase the vital power, and local to break up the membranous deposit in the throat and check the ulcerative process, which might be only partially effected by the general treatment.

My own plan has been to commence the treatment with the Proto-iod-merc. I. and Bi-Chrom-Potash I. in alternation one or two hours apart according to the severity of the symptoms.

When the membranous deposit begin to appear in the throat, continue the remedies and use a gargle of a mild solution of Alum, Chlorate of Soda or Chlorate of Potash. A teaspoon of either may be dissolved in a half-pint glass two-thirds full of water and the throat gargled with it three or four times a day. With little children the throat can be touched gently, with a soft swab, but every thing like harshness should be avoided. Another gargle I have often used with marked benefit, has been, Nitrate of Silver two grains in a glass a third full of water, prepared fresh whenever used. A favorite gargle with me is the disinfecting fluid, which is a solution of chlorate of Soda, one part to ten of water. If, notwithstanding the above treatment, the disease advances, the strength rapidly declines, and there are indications of deep seated ulcerations, the sheet anchor and almost specific, is ARSENICUM, given every hour or two hours. From the first, keep up the strength with nourishing food, such as broth, beef tea, and when the strength is rapidly failing, with wine-whey or milk-punch. During the formation of the membrane, keep the air in the room moist with the vapor of boiling water. It has a softening effect and favors the breaking up and expulsion of the membrane.

But after the disease is apparently cured, after every throat trouble has disappeared and the appetite returned, still watch the patient carefully for two weeks or you may have developed HEART DISEASE, ALBUMINOUS URINE or other troubles. The ALBUMINOUS URINE can be detected by boiling a little of the water, when, if albumen be present, it can be seen in white flakes. The heart trouble, which almost always exists in connection with albuminous urine, and sometimes without it, may be detected by palpitation and oppression of breathing. The remedy in both cases is MERCURIUS.

Diphtheria is not confined to any age, although more prevalent between one and fifteen years of age. It prevails as an epidemic, but I do not look upon it as contagious.

PRICE LIST

OF

MEDICINE CASES FOR FAMILY USE.

One case	(flat) 27 remedies, 1 dr. vials, with book, Dr. Oehme,	$4.25
do.	(upright) lock and key, 40 rem., 1 dr. v., with book, Dr. Tarbells Hom. simplified,..................................	6.00
do.	(upright) lock and key, 65 rem., 1 dr. v., with book, Dr. Hering Domestic Physician, ...	8.00
do.	(upright) lock and key, 78 rem., 1 dr. v., with book, Dr. Pulte Domestic Physician, ...	9.00
do.	(upright) lock and key, 78 rem., 1 dr. v., with book, Dr. Guernsey, or Dr. Hering germ. edition,...........	9.00
do.	(upright) lock and key, 86 rem., 1 dr. v., with book, Dr. Small Dom. Practice, ...	10.00
do.	(upright) lock and key, 80 r. in Globules, 1 dr v., 21 r. in Tinctures, 3 dr. v., with book, Dr. Small, engl. or german, ...	12.00
do.	(upright) lock and key, 104 r., 2 dr. v., with book, suitable to any Domestic Physician,......................	12.00

☞ **A liberal discount will be allowed to the trade.**

Hitchmann, Dr. W. Consumption, its nature, prevention and Homœopathic Treatment, with Illustrations of Homœopathic Practice. Bound,............ 75

Moore, Dr. James. Veterinary Homœopathy, illustrated by 125 cases with Observations,............ 20

Moore, Dr. James. Outlines of Veterinary Homœopathy, comprising Horse, Cow, Dog, Sheep and Hog Diseases, and their Homœopathic Treatment, 2d ed.,............ 1 50

Neidhard, Dr. C. On the Efficacy of Crotalus Horridus in Yellow Fever. Also in Malignant, Bilious and Remittant Fevers. Bound,............ 75

Norton, Dr. J. Edw. Homœopathic Family Medicine,......... 75

Peters, Dr. John C. The Science and Art, or the Principles and Practice of Medicine. Issued in numbers of 96 pages each ; the whole work may reach 21 numbers. On hand No. 1 to 5. Price of each number,............ 50

Physician's Visiting List and Pocket Repertory for 1861,

For 30 patients,............ 1 00

For 60 " 1 20

For 90 " 1 50

The Sixteen Principal Homœopathic Medicines for Family use,............ 45

Ten Reasons for Preferring Homœopathy to the Common System of Medical Treatment.

U. S. Journal of Homœopathy. 1st vol., bound,............ 3 50

☞All other works on Homœopathy in the English, German and French languages always on hand and for sale at publishers prices.

German Books.

Altschul, Dr. J. Systematisches Lehrbuch der theoretischen und praktischen Homöopathie, geb............ $2 00

Argenti, Dr. D. Homöopathische Behandlung verschiedener Krankheiten, mit einer Lebensbeschreibung Hahnemann's. Aus dem Ungarischen übersetzt von Dr. Schleicher, 484 Seiten, geb..... 2 50

Hering, Dr. C. Homöopathischer Hausarzt. 11te Auflage, sehr viel vermehrt und verbessert, geb. $1 5

☞ Mit Arzneikästchen von $8—10.

Hirschel, Dr. Bernhard. Der Homöopathische Arzneischatz in seiner Anwendung am Krankenbette. Für Familie und Haus. 2te Auflage, ... 1

Löwe, Dr. Arthur. Der Homöopathische Kinderarzt. Ein Taschenbuch für Mütter, ...

Lutze, Dr. Arthur. Lehrbuch der Homöopathie für Familiengebrauch. Vollständig, geb. 2

Possart, Dr. A. Homöopathische Arzneimittellehre aller in den Jahren 1858 und 1859 geprüften Mittel nebst Nachträgen aus früheren Jahren, geb. 2

Weber, Dr. J. Der Homöopathische Hausdoktor für Stadt und Land, ...

Wolf, Dr. C. W. Homöopathische Erfahrungen. Die Grundvergiftungen der Menschheit und ihre Befreiung davon, 2—5tes Heft, ... 1

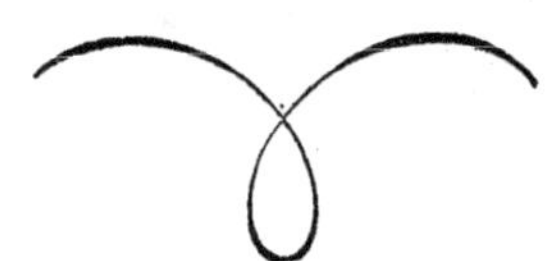

www.ingramcontent.com/pod-product-compliance
Lightning Source LLC
LaVergne TN
LVHW020640110826
845149LV00004B/1299

* 9 7 8 1 4 1 8 1 9 0 6 0 6 *